DR PATRICK WISEDOC

Mastering Ankylosing Spondylitis:

A Comprehensive Guide to Life with AS

"The journey of a thousand miles begins with a single step."

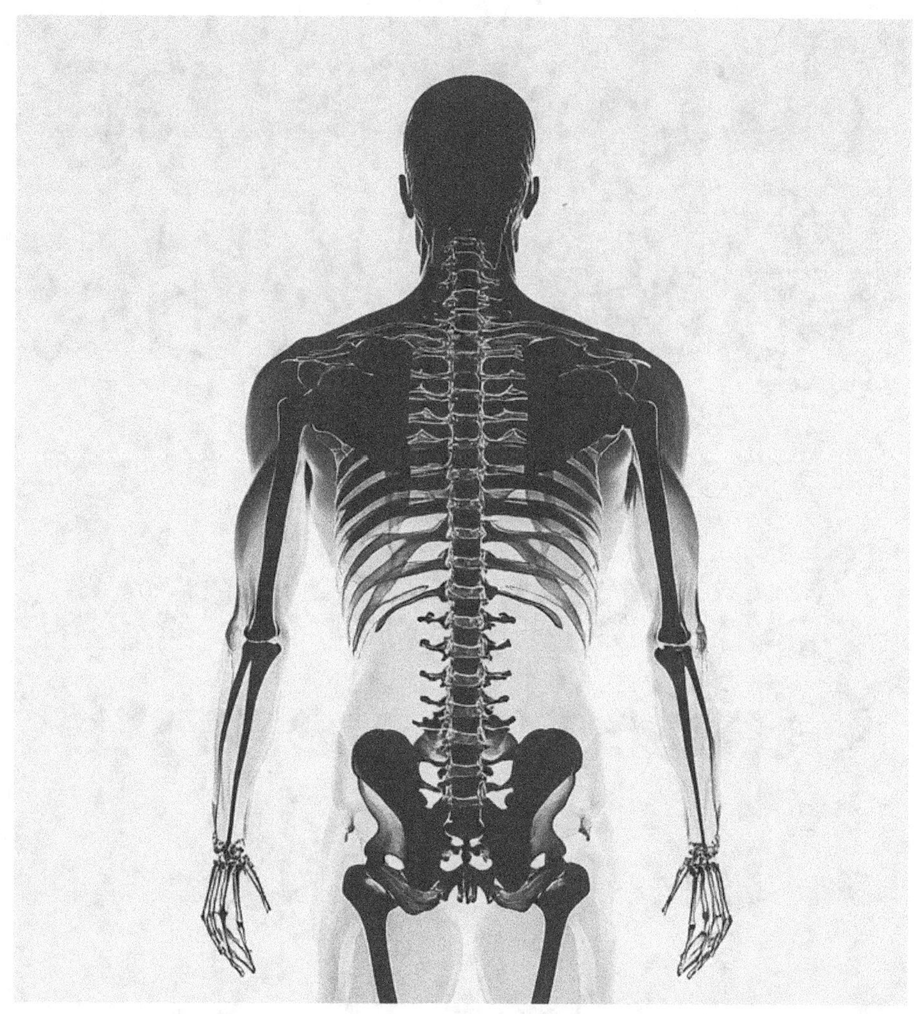

Introduction

Living with Ankylosing Spondylitis (AS) can feel like navigating a complex maze, filled with pain, stiffness, and uncertainty. This comprehensive guide offers a beacon of hope for those seeking to understand and manage this chronic condition.

Mastering Ankylosing Spondylitis : A Comprehensive Guide to Life with AS, is your roadmap to reclaiming control over your life. Delve into the depths of the disease, discover effective strategies for pain management, and explore holistic approaches to healing. From understanding the latest medical advancements to implementing practical lifestyle changes, this book empowers you to take charge of your journey.

Prepare to embark on a transformative path as you unlock the secrets to living a fulfilling life with AS.

Contents

Contents

Contents

Part I: Understanding Ankylosing Spondylitis

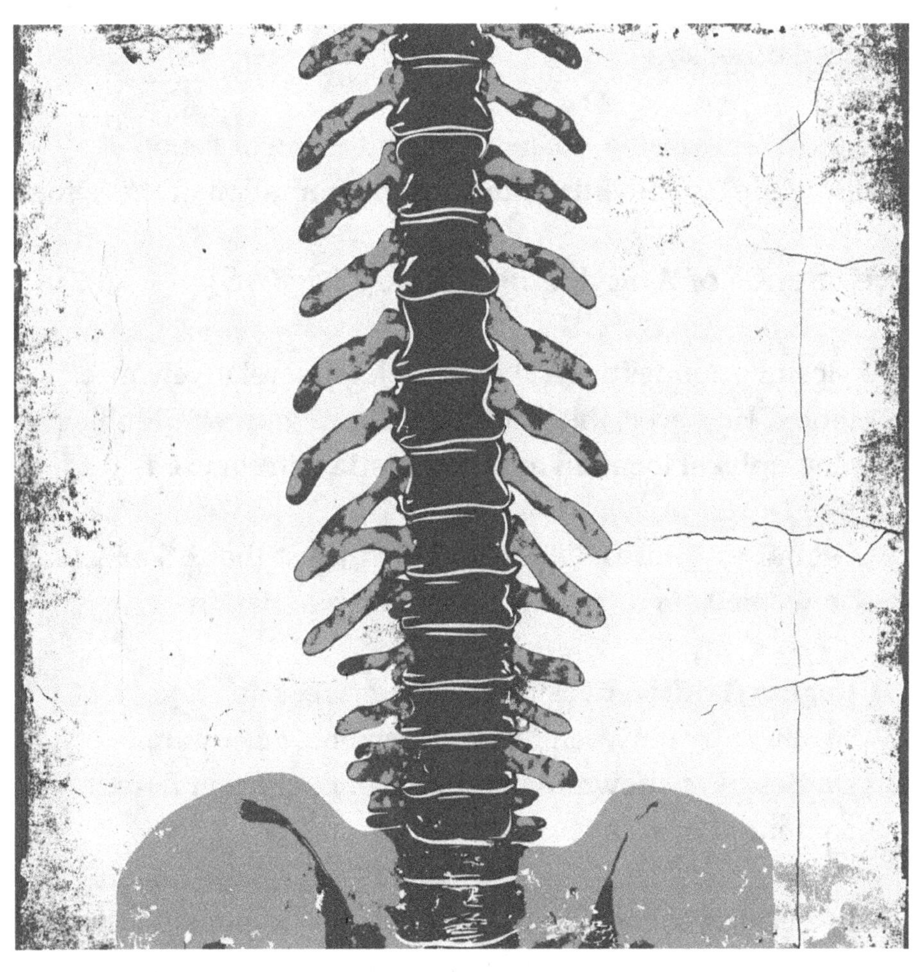

Part I: Understanding Ankylosing Spondylitis
Chapter 1: What is Ankylosing Spondylitis?
Definition, prevalence, and impact

Ankylosing Spondylitis (AS)

Ankylosing spondylitis (AS) is a chronic inflammatory disease primarily affecting the spine. It causes inflammation of the joints in the spine, particularly where the spine meets the pelvis (sacroiliac joints). Over time, this inflammation can lead to the fusion of the vertebrae, resulting in stiffness and reduced mobility.

The term "ankylosing" refers to the stiffening or fusion of joints, while "spondylitis" indicates inflammation of the spine.

Prevalence of Ankylosing Spondylitis (AS)

Ankylosing spondylitis (AS) is considered a relatively rare condition. However, the exact prevalence varies depending on geographical location and diagnostic criteria used.

- **Global estimates:** Older studies suggest that AS affects between 0.1% to 1.4% of the global population.

- **Regional differences:** Prevalence rates can vary significantly between different regions. For example, studies have shown higher prevalence rates in Europe compared to Asia and Africa.

- **Increasing recognition:** It's important to note that the prevalence of AS might be underestimated due to challenges in diagnosis and awareness.

The Impact of Ankylosing Spondylitis (AS)

Ankylosing spondylitis (AS) can significantly impact a person's quality of life. The effects can be both physical and emotional.

Physical Impact

- **Pain and stiffness:** Chronic pain in the spine and other joints is a common symptom, often leading to difficulty with daily activities.

- **Reduced mobility:** As the disease progresses, the spine can become fused, limiting flexibility and causing postural changes.

- **Fatigue:** Many people with AS experience persistent tiredness, affecting energy levels and daily functioning.

- **Other joint involvement:** Inflammation can occur in joints outside the spine, such as the hips, shoulders, and knees.

- **Extra-articular manifestations:** AS can affect other organs, including the eyes (uveitis), heart, lungs, and intestines.

Part I: Understanding Ankylosing Spondylitis
Chapter 1: What is Ankylosing Spondylitis?
Definition, prevalence, and impact

Emotional Impact

- **Depression and anxiety**: The chronic nature of the disease can lead to emotional distress.

- **Body image issues**: Changes in posture and physical appearance can affect self-esteem.

- **Social isolation**: Pain and fatigue can limit social activities and interactions.

It's important to note that the impact of AS varies greatly from person to person. Early diagnosis and management can help to minimize the disease's effects.

Part I: Understanding Ankylosing Spondylitis
Chapter 2: The Anatomy of the Spine
A basic understanding of the spinal column

Structure of the Spine

The spine is a complex structure composed of 33 individual bones called vertebrae. These vertebrae are stacked on top of each other to form the spinal column, which provides support for the body and protects the delicate spinal cord.

The spine is divided into five main sections:

- **Cervical spine:** The upper seven vertebrae, supporting the head and neck.

- **Thoracic spine:** The middle 12 vertebrae, connected to the ribs.

- **Lumbar spine:** The lower five vertebrae, supporting the upper body.

- **Sacrum:** Five fused vertebrae forming the base of the spine.

- **Coccyx:** The tailbone, consisting of several fused vertebrae.

Part I: Understanding Ankylosing Spondylitis
Chapter 2: The Anatomy of the Spine
A basic understanding of the spinal column

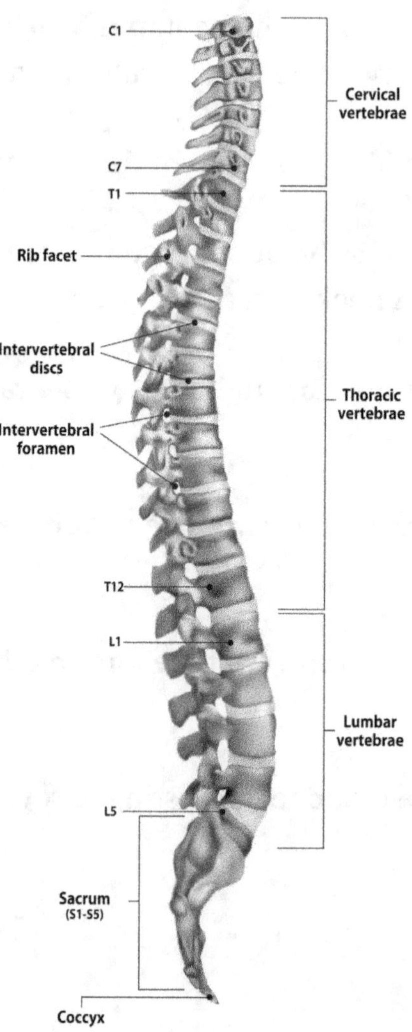

Components of a Vertebra

Each vertebra has several key components:

- **Body**: The main, weight-bearing part of the vertebra.
- **Vertebral arch:** Protects the spinal cord.
- **Spinous process:** A bony projection that can be felt as bumps along the back.
- **Transverse processes**: Extensions of the vertebrae to which muscles and ligaments attach.
- **Intervertebral discs:** Cushioned pads between vertebrae that absorb shock.

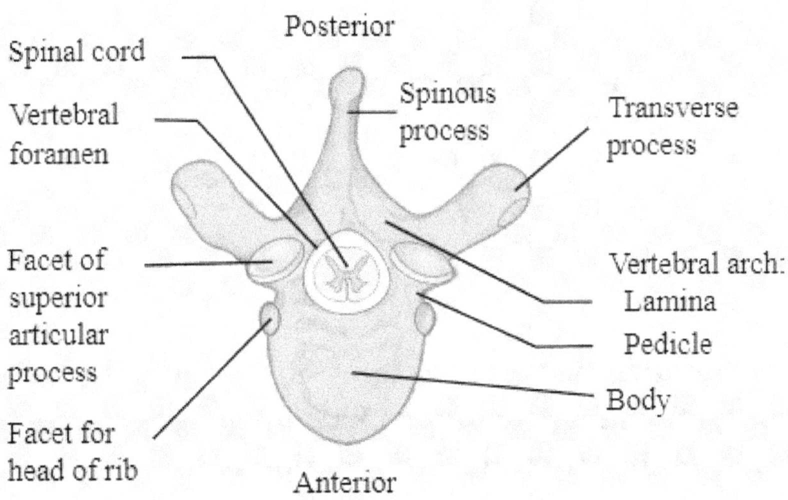

Spinal Curves

The spine is not straight; it has natural curves that help distribute weight and absorb shock. These curves include:

- Cervical lordosis: The inward curve of the neck.
- Thoracic kyphosis: The outward curve of the upper back.
- Lumbar lordosis: The inward curve of the lower back.

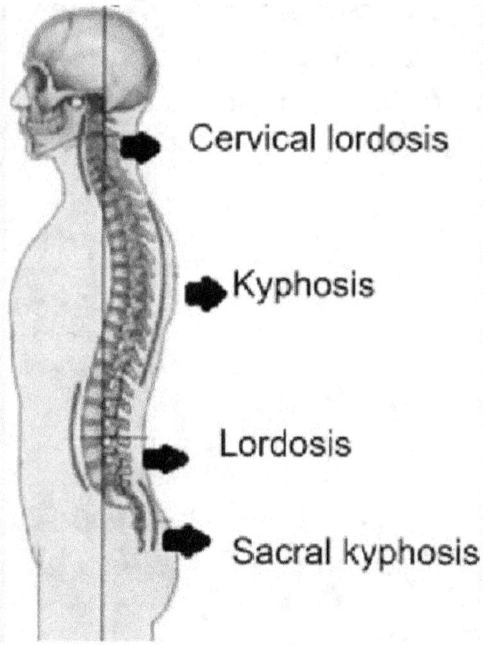

Understanding the basic anatomy of the spine is crucial for comprehending conditions like ankylosing spondylitis, as it affects the structure and function of this vital part of the body.

Part I: Understanding Ankylosing Spondylitis
Chapter 3: The Pathophysiology of Ankylosing Spondylitis
How AS affects the body

Ankylosing spondylitis (AS) is a complex autoimmune disease characterized by chronic inflammation primarily affecting the spine. While the exact cause remains elusive, a combination of genetic and environmental factors is believed to contribute to its development.

Key Players in AS Pathophysiology

- Genetic Predisposition: The HLA-B27 gene is strongly associated with AS. However, it's essential to note that having this gene doesn't automatically mean developing the disease.

- Immune System Dysregulation: In AS, the immune system mistakenly attacks healthy tissues, particularly in the joints. This leads to a chronic inflammatory response.

- Enthesitis: This is a hallmark of AS. It's the inflammation of the entheses, which are the points where tendons and ligaments attach to bone. This inflammation is often the initial stage of the disease.

- Gut Microbiome: Emerging research suggests a link between the gut microbiome and AS. Certain gut bacteria might trigger an immune response in susceptible individuals.

Part I: Understanding Ankylosing Spondylitis
Chapter 3: The Pathophysiology of Ankylosing Spondylitis
How AS affects the body

Disease Progression

- Early Inflammation: The disease typically begins with inflammation in the sacroiliac joints, where the spine connects to the pelvis.

- Enthesitis: Inflammation spreads to other entheses throughout the body, including the spine, shoulders, hips, and heels.

- Bone Formation: As the inflammation persists, the body attempts to repair the damaged tissue by forming new bone. This process, called ossification, can lead to the fusion of vertebrae, resulting in the characteristic "bamboo spine" appearance.

- Extra-Articular Manifestations: In some cases, AS can affect organs outside the musculoskeletal system, including the eyes (uveitis), heart, lungs, and kidneys.

Part I: Understanding Ankylosing Spondylitis
Chapter 3: The Pathophysiology of Ankylosing Spondylitis
How AS affects the body

Inflammatory Cascade

The exact mechanisms underlying the inflammatory process in AS are still being investigated, but it involves a complex interplay of immune cells and inflammatory mediators. Key players include:

- T cells: These immune cells play a central role in initiating and sustaining the inflammatory response.

- Cytokines: These signaling molecules promote inflammation and tissue damage.

- Matrix metalloproteinases (MMPs): These enzymes break down connective tissue, contributing to joint destruction.

Impact on Quality of Life

The chronic inflammation and progressive joint damage associated with AS can significantly impact a person's quality of life. Pain, stiffness, fatigue, and reduced mobility are common symptoms. Additionally, the psychological burden of living with a chronic condition can be substantial.

Understanding the pathophysiology of AS is crucial for developing effective treatment strategies and improving the lives of patients.

Part I: Understanding Ankylosing Spondylitis
Chapter 4: Diagnosis of Ankylosing Spondylitis
Criteria, tests (including radiology, MRI, CT), and
differential diagnosis

Diagnosing Ankylosing Spondylitis (AS) can be challenging as symptoms often mimic other conditions. A combination of clinical criteria, blood tests, and imaging studies is typically used to confirm the diagnosis.

Diagnostic Criteria

The Assessment of Spondyloarthritis International Society (ASAS) has established criteria for diagnosing axial spondyloarthritis (SpA), which includes AS. These criteria consider factors such as:

- Back pain: Chronic lower back pain lasting at least three months that improves with exercise and not with rest.

- Limited lumbar spine mobility: Reduced flexibility in the lower back.

- Limited chest expansion: Decreased ability to expand the chest compared to normal for age and sex.

Blood Tests

While not diagnostic on their own, blood tests can provide valuable information:

- Inflammation markers: Elevated levels of C-reactive protein (CRP) and erythrocyte sedimentation rate (ESR) indicate inflammation in the body.

- HLA-B27 gene: This gene is present in a high percentage of people with AS, but it's not specific to the disease.

Imaging Studies

Imaging tests help visualize changes in the spine and sacroiliac joints:

- X-rays: Can show signs of inflammation and bone fusion in the sacroiliac joints and spine, but early-stage changes might not be visible.

- MRI: More sensitive than X-rays, MRI can detect early inflammation and bone marrow edema.

- CT scans: Provide detailed images of the bones and can be helpful in assessing spinal fusion.

Differential Diagnosis

Several other conditions can mimic the symptoms of AS, making accurate diagnosis essential. Some of these conditions include:

- Mechanical back pain
- Fibromyalgia
- Psoriatic arthritis
- Reactive arthritis
- Inflammatory bowel disease

A thorough medical history, physical examination, and additional tests may be necessary to rule out these conditions and establish a definitive diagnosis of AS.

It's important to note that early diagnosis and treatment of AS can help manage symptoms and prevent disease progression.

Part I: Understanding Ankylosing Spondylitis
Chapter 5: Spondyloarthritis: A Broader Perspective
Relationship between AS and other forms of spondyloarthritis

Spondyloarthritis (SpA) is an umbrella term for a group of inflammatory arthritis conditions that primarily affect the spine and sacroiliac joints. Ankylosing spondylitis (AS) is one of the most well-known types of SpA.

Relationship Between AS and Other Forms of SpA

While AS is a primary form of SpA, there are other related conditions that share similar characteristics. These include:

- Psoriatic arthritis: This condition affects people with psoriasis, a skin condition. Joint inflammation, including in the spine, is a common feature.

- Reactive arthritis: Triggered by an infection, often in the gut or urinary tract, reactive arthritis can cause joint inflammation, including in the spine.

- Enteropathic arthritis: Associated with inflammatory bowel diseases like Crohn's disease and ulcerative colitis, this type of arthritis can also involve the spine.

- Undifferentiated spondyloarthritis: This term is used when the specific type of SpA cannot be definitively diagnosed but the symptoms align with the overall category.

Overlapping Features

These different forms of SpA share several common characteristics:

- Axial involvement: Inflammation of the spine and sacroiliac joints.

- Peripheral arthritis: Inflammation in joints outside the spine.

- Enthesitis: Inflammation where tendons and ligaments attach to bone.

- Uveitis: Inflammation of the eye.

- Skin manifestations: Psoriasis or other skin conditions.

While the specific triggers and underlying mechanisms may vary between different types of SpA, there are overlapping features that suggest a common underlying pathophysiology.

Understanding the relationship between AS and other forms of SpA is essential for accurate diagnosis and appropriate management.

A Deeper Dive into Spondyloarthritis

Understanding the Different Forms of SpA
Let's explore the specific characteristics and challenges
associated with each type of SpA:

Ankylosing Spondylitis (AS)

- Primary focus: Inflammation of the spine and sacroiliac
  joints.

- Characteristic symptoms: Back pain, stiffness, reduced
  spinal mobility, fatigue.

- Extra-articular manifestations: Uveitis, inflammatory
  bowel disease, heart, lung, and kidney involvement.

Psoriatic Arthritis (PsA)

- Connection to psoriasis: Often develops in individuals
  with psoriasis, a skin condition.

- Joint involvement: Can affect any joint, including the
  spine, but often presents with symmetrical joint swelling.

- Other symptoms: Nail changes, skin inflammation, and
  eye inflammation can occur.

Part I: Understanding Ankylosing Spondylitis
Chapter 5: Spondyloarthritis: A Broader Perspective
Relationship between AS and other forms of spondyloarthritis

Reactive Arthritis (ReA)

- Trigger: Often follows an infection, such as a urinary tract infection or gastrointestinal infection.

- Joint involvement: Can affect multiple joints, including the spine.

- Other symptoms: Eye inflammation (uveitis), skin rash (erythema nodosum), and mouth ulcers.

Enteropathic Arthritis

- Associated with: Inflammatory bowel diseases like Crohn's disease and ulcerative colitis.

- Joint involvement: Can affect any joint, including the spine.

- Other symptoms: Digestive issues related to the underlying inflammatory bowel disease.

Undifferentiated Spondyloarthritis

- Complex presentation: Symptoms overlap with other forms of SpA, making it difficult to pinpoint a specific diagnosis.

- Management: Treatment focuses on managing symptoms and preventing disease progression.

Relationship between AS and other forms of spondyloarthritis

Overlapping Features and Challenges

While each type of SpA has unique characteristics, they share common challenges:

- Chronic pain and fatigue: These are often debilitating symptoms affecting daily life.

- Reduced mobility: Joint stiffness and inflammation can limit physical activity.

- Psychological impact: The chronic nature of the disease can lead to depression, anxiety, and isolation.

- Diagnostic challenges: Differentiating between different forms of SpA can be complex, requiring careful evaluation.

Part I: Understanding Ankylosing Spondylitis
Chapter 5: Spondyloarthritis: A Broader Perspective
Relationship between AS and other forms of spondyloarthritis

Treatment Approaches

Treatment for SpA is tailored to the specific type and severity of the disease. Common approaches include:

- Medications: Nonsteroidal anti-inflammatory drugs (NSAIDs), corticosteroids, disease-modifying antirheumatic drugs (DMARDs), and biologic agents.

- Physical therapy: Exercises to improve flexibility, strength, and posture.

- Lifestyle modifications: Weight management, regular exercise, and stress reduction.

Part II: Living with Ankylosing Spondylitis

Part II: Living with Ankylosing Spondylitis
Chapter 6: Early Symptoms and Recognition
Identifying potential signs of AS

Early detection of Ankylosing Spondylitis (AS) is crucial for effective management. Unfortunately, the initial symptoms can be subtle and often mistaken for other conditions.

Common Early Symptoms

- Back pain: This is the most common initial symptom. It's often described as a dull, aching pain in the lower back, especially in the morning or after periods of inactivity.

- Stiffness: Morning stiffness is characteristic of AS. It may improve with activity but returns after periods of rest.

- Fatigue: Feeling tired and exhausted even with adequate sleep is a common early symptom.

- Reduced range of motion: Difficulty bending forward or twisting the spine can be an early indicator.

Less Common Early Symptoms

- Pain in other joints: While primarily a spinal condition, AS can also affect other joints like shoulders, hips, and knees.

- Eye inflammation (uveitis): This can cause redness, pain, and blurred vision.

- Psoriasis: A skin condition characterized by red, scaly patches.

- Inflammatory bowel disease (IBD): Conditions like Crohn's disease or ulcerative colitis can occur in people with AS.

Recognizing the Signs

It's essential to pay attention to these symptoms and consult a healthcare professional if they persist or worsen. Early diagnosis and treatment can significantly improve the quality of life for individuals with AS.

Remember: While these symptoms are common in AS, they can also be associated with other conditions. A healthcare professional will conduct a thorough evaluation to determine the underlying cause.

Deeper Dive into Early AS Symptoms

While we've covered the primary early symptoms of Ankylosing Spondylitis (AS), it's essential to understand the nuances and potential variations.

Back Pain Characteristics

- Location: Typically begins in the lower back (lumbar spine) but can spread to the upper back (thoracic spine).
- Nature: Often described as a deep, aching pain that worsens with rest and improves with activity.
- Pattern: May fluctuate in intensity, but generally tends to worsen over time.

Stiffness

- Morning stiffness: Characteristically pronounced upon waking and gradually improves throughout the day.
- Joint stiffness: Stiffness can also affect other joints, such as the shoulders, hips, and knees.

Fatigue

- Nature: Often described as a persistent, overwhelming tiredness that doesn't improve with rest.
- Impact: Can significantly affect daily activities and quality of life.

Less Common but Important Symptoms

- Uveitis: Inflammation of the eye can cause pain, redness, blurred vision, and sensitivity to light.
- Heel pain: Inflammation at the attachment of the Achilles tendon can cause heel pain.
- Chest pain: In some cases, inflammation of the costovertebral joints (where ribs attach to the spine) can cause chest pain.

Recognizing Patterns

It's crucial to observe symptom patterns. If you experience:

- Gradual onset of back pain
- Morning stiffness
- Fatigue
- Limited spinal mobility

Over a period of weeks or months, it's essential to consult a healthcare professional.

Remember: Early diagnosis and treatment are key to managing AS effectively.

Pain and fatigue are common challenges for individuals with Ankylosing Spondylitis (AS). While these symptoms can be debilitating, effective management strategies can significantly improve quality of life.

Pain Management Strategies

- Medication: Nonsteroidal anti-inflammatory drugs (NSAIDs), corticosteroids, and disease-modifying antirheumatic drugs (DMARDs) can help reduce inflammation and pain.

- Heat and cold therapy: Applying heat or cold packs to the affected areas can provide temporary relief.

- Physical therapy: Exercises designed to improve flexibility, strength, and posture can help manage pain.

- Pain management techniques: Relaxation techniques like meditation, deep breathing, and yoga can help cope with pain.

Part II: Living with Ankylosing Spondylitis
Chapter 7: Managing Pain and Fatigue
Strategies for coping with common AS symptoms

Fatigue Management Strategies

- Pacing activities: Balancing rest and activity is essential. Breaking tasks into smaller, manageable steps can help prevent fatigue.

- Prioritizing tasks: Focusing on essential activities and delegating or eliminating less important tasks can conserve energy.

- Regular exercise: While it may seem counterintuitive, regular physical activity can improve energy levels and reduce fatigue in the long term.

- Healthy sleep: Ensuring adequate sleep is crucial for managing fatigue. Establishing a consistent sleep routine can help.

- Energy conservation techniques: Identifying energy-saving strategies, such as using assistive devices or avoiding unnecessary physical exertion, can help manage fatigue.

Combining Strategies

It's important to find a combination of strategies that works best for you. A multi-faceted approach often yields the best results. Regular communication with your healthcare provider is essential to develop an effective management plan.

Part II: Living with Ankylosing Spondylitis
Chapter 8: Exercise and Physical Therapy
The importance of physical activity and specific recommendations

Exercise and Physical Therapy for Ankylosing Spondylitis (AS)

Regular physical activity is a cornerstone of managing Ankylosing Spondylitis (AS). It helps maintain flexibility, strength, and overall well-being. Working with a physical therapist can provide tailored exercises and guidance.

The Importance of Exercise

- Pain management: Regular movement can help reduce stiffness and pain.

- Improved mobility: Exercises can help maintain and improve range of motion in the spine and other joints.

- Increased strength: Building muscle strength can support the spine and alleviate pressure on joints.

- Enhanced posture: Proper exercises can help correct postural issues and reduce strain on the spine.

- Boosted mood: Physical activity can improve mental health and overall well-being.

Types of Exercises

- Flexibility exercises: Stretching helps maintain joint mobility and reduce stiffness. Examples include hamstring stretches, hip flexor stretches, and spinal twists.

- Strengthening exercises: Building muscle strength supports the spine and improves stability. Exercises like planks, bridges, and shoulder blade squeezes can be beneficial.

- Aerobic exercises: Low-impact activities like swimming, cycling, or walking can improve cardiovascular health and overall fitness.

- Water-based exercises: The buoyancy of water can reduce joint stress while providing resistance for muscle strengthening.

Part II: Living with Ankylosing Spondylitis
Chapter 8: Exercise and Physical Therapy
The importance of physical activity and specific recommendations

Specific Recommendations

- Consult a physical therapist: A qualified professional can create a personalized exercise plan based on your specific needs and limitations.

- Listen to your body: It's essential to avoid pain and overexertion.

- Consistency: Regular exercise is key to achieving long-term benefits.

- Warm-up and cool-down: Incorporate these into your routine to prevent injuries.

- Incorporate relaxation techniques: Combining exercise with relaxation techniques like deep breathing can enhance the overall experience.

Remember, the goal is to find exercises that you enjoy and can incorporate into your daily routine. Regular physical activity, along with other management strategies, can significantly improve your quality of life with AS.

Individuals with Ankylosing Spondylitis (AS) are at a higher risk of developing osteoporosis, a condition that weakens bones. This is due to several factors, including chronic inflammation, reduced mobility, and certain medications used to treat AS.

Building Stronger Bones

To help prevent osteoporosis and maintain bone density, consider these steps:

- Weight-bearing exercises: These exercises put stress on your bones, stimulating them to become stronger. Examples include walking, jogging, dancing, and climbing stairs.

- Strength training: Building muscle mass can indirectly support bone health. Exercises like lifting weights or using resistance bands can be beneficial.

- Calcium and Vitamin D: These nutrients are essential for bone health. Incorporate dairy products (milk, yogurt, cheese), leafy green vegetables (kale, spinach), and fortified foods (orange juice, cereal) into your diet.

- Regular check-ups: Consult your doctor about bone density screenings and discuss any concerns about bone health.

Lifestyle Factors

- Limit alcohol and smoking: Both can negatively impact bone health.
- Fall prevention: Take steps to prevent falls, as fractures can be more severe in people with osteoporosis.
- Balanced diet: Ensure you're consuming a variety of foods to support overall health and bone strength.

The Importance of Weight-Bearing Exercise

As mentioned, weight-bearing exercises are crucial for bone health. These exercises involve working against gravity, placing stress on your bones, and stimulating new bone growth.

- Examples: Walking, jogging, dancing, hiking, and stair climbing.

- Intensity: Aim for at least 30 minutes of moderate-intensity weight-bearing exercise most days of the week.

- Consult your doctor: Before starting any new exercise regimen, consult with your healthcare provider to determine what is safe and appropriate for your condition.

Part II: Living with Ankylosing Spondylitis
Chapter 9: Bone Health and Ankylosing Spondylitis
Preventing osteoporosis and maintaining bone density

Strength Training

Building muscle mass can indirectly support bone health. Strength training exercises also improve balance and coordination, reducing the risk of falls.

- Examples: Lifting weights, using resistance bands, bodyweight exercises like squats, lunges, and push-ups.

- Frequency: Aim for strength training exercises at least twice a week.

- Progression: Gradually increase the weight or resistance as you get stronger.

Nutrition for Bone Health

A balanced diet rich in calcium and vitamin D is essential for strong bones.

- Calcium-rich foods: Dairy products (milk, yogurt, cheese), leafy green vegetables (kale, spinach, broccoli), fortified plant-based milk, tofu, and almonds.

- Vitamin D-rich foods: Fatty fish (salmon, tuna), egg yolks, fortified dairy products, and fortified cereals.

- Vitamin D supplements: Your doctor may recommend a vitamin D supplement, especially if you have limited sun exposure.

Additional Tips

- Hydration: Drinking plenty of water is essential for overall health, including bone health.

- Regular check-ups: Schedule regular check-ups with your healthcare provider to monitor your bone health and discuss any concerns.

- Fall prevention: Take steps to reduce the risk of falls, such as removing clutter, using assistive devices if needed, and improving lighting.

By incorporating these strategies into your daily routine, you can significantly improve your bone health and reduce the risk of osteoporosis. Remember, it's essential to listen to your body and consult with your healthcare provider for personalized guidance.

Making adjustments to your daily routine can significantly improve your quality of life with Ankylosing Spondylitis (AS). Here are some key lifestyle modifications:

Prioritizing Sleep

- Consistent sleep schedule: Try to go to bed and wake up at the same time each day.
- Sleep environment: Create a calm and dark sleep environment.
- Limit screen time: Reduce exposure to screens before bed.

Managing Stress

- Stress reduction techniques: Practice relaxation techniques like meditation, deep breathing, or yoga.
- Time management: Prioritize tasks and avoid overcommitting yourself.
- Support system: Build a strong support network of friends, family, or support groups.

Maintaining a Healthy Weight

- Balanced diet: Focus on whole foods, fruits, vegetables, and lean proteins.
- Portion control: Be mindful of portion sizes to maintain a healthy weight.
- Regular physical activity: Exercise can help manage weight and improve overall health.

Part II: Living with Ankylosing Spondylitis
Chapter 10: Lifestyle Modifications
Adapting daily life to manage AS

Ergonomic Considerations

- Workspace setup: Ensure your workspace is ergonomically designed to prevent strain.
- Proper posture: Maintain good posture while sitting, standing, and sleeping.
- Regular breaks: Take short breaks to stretch and move around.

Heat and Cold Therapy

- Heat application: Can help relieve muscle stiffness and pain.
- Cold therapy: Can reduce inflammation and numb pain.

Regular Check-ups

- Monitor symptoms: Keep track of your symptoms and discuss any changes with your healthcare provider.
- Adherence to treatment: Follow your doctor's prescribed treatment plan.
- Early intervention: Address any concerns or flare-ups promptly.

Support Groups

- Connect with others: Sharing experiences with people who understand can be beneficial.
- Emotional support: Support groups provide emotional support and coping strategies.

Lifestyle Modifications: A Deeper Dive

Prioritizing Sleep: The Foundation for Well-being
Adequate sleep is crucial for managing AS symptoms.

- Sleep hygiene: Establish a relaxing bedtime routine, create a sleep-conducive environment (dark, quiet, cool), and avoid stimulants before bed.

- Sleep aids: If sleep disturbances persist, consult your doctor about potential sleep aids.

- Nap time: Short naps during the day can be beneficial for managing fatigue, but avoid long naps that disrupt nighttime sleep.

Managing Stress: Finding Balance

Chronic stress can exacerbate AS symptoms.

- Stress management techniques: Incorporate relaxation techniques like meditation, deep breathing, or progressive muscle relaxation into your daily routine.

- Time management: Prioritize tasks, delegate when possible, and learn to say no to overwhelming commitments.

- Support system: Build a strong support network of friends, family, or support groups.

Maintaining a Healthy Weight: The Benefits Beyond Appearance

Weight management is essential for overall health and can positively impact AS symptoms.

- Balanced diet: Focus on whole foods, fruits, vegetables, lean proteins, and whole grains.

- Portion control: Be mindful of portion sizes to avoid overeating.

- Regular physical activity: Aim for a balance of cardiovascular exercise, strength training, and flexibility exercises.

- Consult a dietitian: If needed, seek guidance from a registered dietitian to create a personalized meal plan.

Ergonomic Considerations: Creating a Comfortable Environment

Adjusting your environment can significantly impact your comfort and function.

- Workspace setup: Ensure your chair, desk, and computer monitor are at the correct height to maintain good posture.
- Supportive seating: Invest in a supportive chair with lumbar support.

- Regular breaks: Get up and move around every 30 minutes to prevent stiffness.

Heat and Cold Therapy: Tailoring Relief

- Heat therapy: Apply heat packs or take warm baths to relax muscles and relieve stiffness.

- Cold therapy: Use ice packs to reduce inflammation and numb pain in flare-ups.

- Experimentation: Determine which method works best for you and when.

By implementing these lifestyle modifications, you can significantly improve your quality of life with AS. Remember, it's essential to listen to your body and make adjustments as needed.

Part II: Living with Ankylosing Spondylitis
Chapter 11: Psychological Well-being
Coping with the emotional impact of AS

Living with a chronic condition like AS can significantly impact emotional well-being. It's essential to acknowledge and address the psychological challenges that come with the disease.

The Emotional Impact of AS

- Depression and anxiety: These are common mental health conditions associated with chronic pain and limited mobility.

- Frustration and anger: Dealing with the unpredictability of symptoms can lead to feelings of frustration and anger.

- Isolation: Feeling disconnected from others due to physical limitations or emotional challenges.

- Body image issues: Changes in appearance or physical limitations can affect self-esteem.

Coping Strategies

- Open communication: Talk to friends, family, or a therapist about your feelings. Sharing your experiences can provide emotional relief.

- Support groups: Connecting with others who understand your condition can offer valuable support and coping strategies.

- Mindfulness and meditation: These practices can help reduce stress and improve overall well-being.

- Setting realistic goals: Break down tasks into smaller, manageable steps to avoid feeling overwhelmed.

- Seeking professional help: If you're struggling to cope, consider seeking help from a mental health professional.

- Physical activity: Regular exercise has been shown to improve mood and reduce stress.

Building Resilience

- Positive thinking: Focus on what you can control and celebrate small victories.

- Time management: Prioritize tasks and allow yourself rest periods.

- Healthy lifestyle: Maintaining a balanced diet, regular exercise, and adequate sleep can contribute to overall well-being.

- Self-care: Make time for activities you enjoy, such as hobbies or spending time in nature.

Remember, it's okay to seek help if you're struggling. By prioritizing your mental health, you can improve your overall quality of life with AS.

Part III: Treatment Options

Chapter 12: Conventional Medical Treatment
Pharmacologic therapies and their role in management

Conventional Medical Treatment for Ankylosing Spondylitis (AS)

Pharmacological treatments play a crucial role in managing Ankylosing Spondylitis (AS) by reducing inflammation, pain, and stiffness. Several classes of medications are used to address different aspects of the disease.

Nonsteroidal Anti-Inflammatory Drugs (NSAIDs)

- First-line treatment: NSAIDs are often the initial treatment due to their effectiveness in reducing pain and inflammation.
- Examples: Ibuprofen, naproxen, diclofenac.

- Benefits: Rapid onset of action, improvement in joint stiffness and pain.

Disease-Modifying Anti-Rheumatic Drugs (DMARDs)

- Slower onset of action: DMARDs work gradually to modify the disease process.
- Examples: Sulfasalazine, methotrexate.
- Benefits: Can help reduce inflammation and slow disease progression.

Part III: Treatment Options
Chapter 12: Conventional Medical Treatment
Pharmacologic therapies and their role in management

Corticosteroids

- Short-term relief: Corticosteroids are used for acute flares or severe symptoms.
- Administration: Can be administered orally, intravenously, or as injections directly into affected joints.
- Side effects: Long-term use can lead to significant side effects, so they are generally used cautiously.

Biological Therapies

- Targeted treatment: These medications target specific immune system proteins involved in inflammation.

- Examples: Tumor necrosis factor (TNF) inhibitors, interleukin-17 (IL-17) inhibitors, Janus kinase (JAK) inhibitors.

- Benefits: Effective in managing severe AS, often leading to significant symptom improvement.

Other Medications

- Bone health: Medications like bisphosphonates may be prescribed to protect bone health.

- Pain management: Opioids are generally avoided due to the risk of addiction, but may be considered in severe, refractory cases.

Important Considerations

- Individualized treatment: The best treatment approach varies from person to person.

- Potential side effects: All medications have potential side effects, and regular monitoring is essential.

- Combination therapy: Often, a combination of medications is used to achieve optimal results.

- Non-pharmacological treatments: Exercise, physical therapy, and lifestyle modifications complement medical treatment.

It's crucial to work closely with your healthcare provider to determine the most appropriate treatment plan for your specific condition

Part III: Treatment Options
Chapter 13: Natural and Complementary Therapies
**Exploring alternative approaches (herbs, Ayurveda,
aromatherapy, meditation, yoga)**

While conventional medicine is essential for managing AS, many people find relief and improved well-being through complementary approaches. Always consult your healthcare provider before starting any new treatment.

Herbs

- Disclaimer: The use of herbs should be approached with caution and under the guidance of a qualified herbalist.
- Some herbs have traditionally been used for their anti-inflammatory properties. However, scientific evidence supporting their effectiveness in AS is limited.

Ayurveda

- This ancient Indian system of medicine focuses on holistic health.
- It involves tailored dietary changes, lifestyle modifications, and herbal remedies based on an individual's constitution.
- Ayurveda emphasizes balance and prevention.

Aromatherapy

- Using essential oils can promote relaxation and stress reduction.
- Lavender and chamomile are often used for their calming properties.
- Aromatherapy can be incorporated through massage, baths, or diffusers.

Part III: Treatment Options
Chapter 13: Natural and Complementary Therapies
Exploring alternative approaches (herbs, Ayurveda, aromatherapy, meditation, yoga)

Meditation and Yoga

- These practices offer numerous benefits for physical and mental well-being.
- Regular meditation can reduce stress and improve focus.
- Gentle forms of yoga, like Hatha or Yin, can increase flexibility and manage pain.

Other Complementary Therapies

- Acupuncture: This involves inserting thin needles into specific points on the body to stimulate energy flow.
- Massage therapy: Can relax muscles, reduce tension, and improve circulation.
- Chiropractic care: Focuses on the musculoskeletal system and may provide relief for some individuals.

Important Considerations

- Individual response: The effectiveness of complementary therapies varies widely.
- Safety: Some herbs and supplements can interact with medications or have side effects.
- Qualified practitioners: Seek practitioners with experience in treating chronic conditions.
- Combination therapy: Complementary therapies often work best in conjunction with conventional treatments.

Exploring alternative approaches (herbs, Ayurveda, aromatherapy, meditation, yoga)

Aromatherapy for Ankylosing Spondylitis (AS)
Aromatherapy involves using essential oils for therapeutic benefits. While there's limited scientific research specifically on aromatherapy for AS, it's often used as a complementary approach to manage symptoms.

How Aromatherapy Might Help

- Pain relief: Some essential oils have analgesic properties that may help reduce pain.
- Stress reduction: Aromatherapy can promote relaxation and reduce stress, which can indirectly alleviate AS symptoms.
- Improved sleep: Certain oils can help improve sleep quality, which is often disrupted in people with AS.

Popular Essential Oils for AS

- Lavender: Known for its calming and relaxing properties.
- Peppermint: May help with pain relief and improved digestion.
- Eucalyptus: Often used for its anti-inflammatory properties.
- Rosemary: Can be stimulating and may help with focus and concentration.

Part III: Treatment Options
Chapter 13: Natural and Complementary Therapies
Exploring alternative approaches (herbs, Ayurveda, aromatherapy, meditation, yoga)

Ways to Use Essential Oils

- Inhalation: Directly inhale the aroma from the bottle or use a diffuser.
- Topical application: Dilute essential oils in a carrier oil (like coconut or jojoba) and apply to the skin.
- Bath: Add a few drops of essential oil to your bathwater.

Important Considerations

- Allergies: Some people may be allergic to essential oils.
- Dilution: Always dilute essential oils before applying them to the skin.
- Pregnancy and breastfeeding: Consult with a healthcare provider before using essential oils during pregnancy or breastfeeding.
- Medical advice: Aromatherapy should be considered a complementary therapy, not a replacement for medical treatment.

While aromatherapy may offer some benefits for people with AS, it's essential to approach it with caution and consult with a healthcare professional if you have any concerns.

Chapter 14: Nutrition and Ankylosing Spondylitis
The role of diet in managing inflammation

While there's no specific diet proven to cure Ankylosing Spondylitis (AS), focusing on anti-inflammatory foods can help manage symptoms.

The Role of Diet in Managing Inflammation

- Anti-inflammatory foods: Incorporate plenty of fruits, vegetables, whole grains, lean proteins, and healthy fats into your diet. These foods contain antioxidants and omega-3 fatty acids, which can help reduce inflammation.

- Omega-3 fatty acids: Found in fatty fish (salmon, mackerel, sardines), flaxseeds, chia seeds, and walnuts, these fats can help reduce joint stiffness and inflammation.

- Limited processed foods: These often contain high levels of unhealthy fats, added sugars, and sodium, which can contribute to inflammation.

- Hydration: Drinking plenty of water helps maintain overall health and can aid digestion.

Part III: Treatment Options
Chapter 14: Nutrition and Ankylosing Spondylitis
The role of diet in managing inflammation

Foods to Emphasize

- Fruits and vegetables: Rich in antioxidants and vitamins.
- Whole grains: Provide fiber and sustained energy.
- Lean proteins: Chicken, fish, beans, and lentils are good options.
- Healthy fats: Found in avocados, nuts, seeds, and olive oil.

Foods to Limit

- Red meat: High in saturated fat, which can contribute to inflammation.
- Processed foods: Often high in unhealthy fats, sodium, and added sugars.
- Refined carbohydrates: White bread, pasta, and sugary drinks can spike blood sugar levels.

Additional Tips

- Portion control: Pay attention to portion sizes to maintain a healthy weight.
- Food diary: Tracking your food intake can help identify potential triggers and patterns.
- Consult a dietitian: A registered dietitian can provide personalized guidance.

Remember, while diet can play a role in managing AS symptoms, it's essential to combine it with other treatment approaches, such as medication and exercise.

Part III: Treatment Options
Chapter 14: Nutrition and Ankylosing Spondylitis
The role of diet in managing inflammation

Foods to Emphasize

- Fruits and vegetables: Rich in antioxidants and vitamins.
- Whole grains: Provide fiber and sustained energy.
- Lean proteins: Chicken, fish, beans, and lentils are good options.
- Healthy fats: Found in avocados, nuts, seeds, and olive oil.

Foods to Limit

- Red meat: High in saturated fat, which can contribute to inflammation.
- Processed foods: Often high in unhealthy fats, sodium, and added sugars.
- Refined carbohydrates: White bread, pasta, and sugary drinks can spike blood sugar levels.

Additional Tips

- Portion control: Pay attention to portion sizes to maintain a healthy weight.
- Food diary: Tracking your food intake can help identify potential triggers and patterns.
- Consult a dietitian: A registered dietitian can provide personalized guidance.

Remember, while diet can play a role in managing AS symptoms, it's essential to combine it with other treatment approaches, such as medication and exercise.

Chapter 15: Surgical Interventions
When and why surgery might be considered

Surgical Interventions for Ankylosing Spondylitis (AS) Surgery is typically considered a last resort for managing Ankylosing Spondylitis (AS) when conservative treatments like medication, physical therapy, and lifestyle modifications have proven ineffective.

Reasons for Surgery

- Severe pain: When pain is debilitating and unresponsive to other treatments.
- Neurological symptoms: If nerve compression is causing numbness, weakness, or tingling.
- Spinal deformity: In cases of severe spinal curvature that impacts daily function or quality of life.
- Joint damage: If hip or shoulder joints are severely damaged and causing significant pain.

Types of Surgery

- Laminectomy: Removes part of the vertebra to relieve pressure on the spinal cord or nerves.
- Spinal fusion: Fuses two or more vertebrae together to stabilize the spine.
- Osteotomy: Involves cutting and repositioning the spine to correct severe curvature.
- Joint replacement: Hip or shoulder replacement may be considered for severe joint damage.

Part III: Treatment Options
Chapter 15: Surgical Interventions
When and why surgery might be considered

Considerations

- Risks: Surgery carries inherent risks, including infection, bleeding, and nerve damage.
- Recovery: Post-surgery recovery can be lengthy and challenging.
- Lifestyle changes: Significant lifestyle adjustments may be necessary after surgery.

Decision-Making

The decision to undergo surgery is a complex one. It involves careful consideration of the potential benefits and risks, as well as discussions with healthcare providers.
It's crucial to explore all conservative treatment options before considering surgery.

Part IV: Support and Resources

Chapter 16: Support Groups and Communities
Connecting with others living with AS

Connecting with others who understand the challenges of living with AS can provide invaluable emotional support and practical advice.

Benefits of Support Groups

- Shared experiences: Connecting with people who face similar challenges can help you feel less alone.
- Coping strategies: Learn from others' experiences and adapt their coping mechanisms.
- Emotional support: Sharing feelings and concerns with others can be therapeutic.
- Information exchange: Stay updated on the latest research and treatment options.
- Advocacy: Join forces to raise awareness and advocate for better support and resources.

Finding a Support Group

- Online communities: Numerous online forums and support groups offer a platform to connect with people worldwide.
- Local organizations: Check with local hospitals, arthritis foundations, or patient advocacy groups for in-person support groups.
- Social media: Use platforms like Facebook and Twitter to find AS support groups and connect with others.

Part IV: Support and Resources
Chapter 16: Support Groups and Communities
Connecting with others living with AS

Building a Supportive Network

- Reach out: Initiate contact with others living with AS, whether online or in person.
- Share your experiences: Be open about your challenges and feelings.
- Active listening: Offer support and encouragement to others.
- Respect boundaries: Understand that everyone's experience with AS is unique.

By actively participating in a support group or community, you can build a strong network of individuals who share your journey and offer understanding, support, and hope.

Chapter 17: Research and Future Directions

Updates on ongoing research and potential breakthroughs

The field of Ankylosing Spondylitis (AS) research is continually evolving, with promising advancements on the horizon.

Current Research Focus

- Understanding the disease: Researchers are delving deeper into the underlying causes of AS, including genetic and environmental factors.

- Novel biomarkers: Identifying biomarkers can aid in early diagnosis and disease monitoring.

- Treatment optimization: Studies are exploring new drug combinations and personalized treatment approaches.

- Quality of life: Research focuses on improving the overall well-being of individuals with AS.

Part IV: Support and Resources
Chapter 17: Research and Future Directions
Updates on ongoing research and potential breakthroughs

Potential Breakthroughs

- Disease-modifying therapies: The development of drugs that can halt or reverse disease progression is a major goal.
- Gene therapy: Targeting specific genes involved in AS could offer new treatment options.
- Regenerative medicine: Stem cell therapy and tissue engineering hold promise for repairing damaged tissues.
- Precision medicine: Tailored treatments based on individual genetic makeup and disease characteristics.

Staying Informed

To stay updated on the latest research:

- Follow reputable medical organizations: Organizations like the Arthritis Foundation and the Spondylitis Association of America provide valuable information.
- Participate in clinical trials: Consider enrolling in clinical trials to contribute to research and potentially benefit from new treatments.
- Connect with online communities: Engage with other patients and researchers to share information and support.

While there's no cure for AS yet, ongoing research brings hope for improved treatments and a better quality of life for those affected.